Chronic Lymphatic Leukemia Remission?

ISBN-13: 978-1976239014
ISBN-10: 197623901X

Courduff Publications
14208 River Oaks Drive
Foley, Alabama 36535

Chronic Lympahtic Leukemia Remission?

Table of Contents

ACKNOWLEDGEMENTS

TO MY DOCTORS:

My thanks to my medical doctors for their professional care over the past 16 years, when my medical journey began with quadruple heart bypass surgery. Up until then, my health had never been a concern for me. I was strong, active, worked day and night, and felt I was on top of the world.

The heart surgery was a major wakeup call. I now take my health seriously. The doctors successfully repaired my heart. I thought my health problems would be under control but one diagnosis remained and created concern and uncertainty and left me feeling out of control.

The complete mystery was the new diagnosis—Chronic Lymphatic Leukemia.

This book is about Chronic Lymphatic Leukemia. There are so many questions, and so few answers when researching the cause and the cure for CLL (Chronic Lymphatic Leukemia).

Thank you, to the many doctors who have taken care of me over the last 16 years. Now my wish is that medical scientists are able to find the cause and a cure for CLL.

INTRODUCTION

Due to my diagnosis, I researched the disease and found very little information about this disease. Most research is written in medical journals that are almost incomprehensible to nonmedical people. We felt there is a need for some basic information and we put together our journey of living and learning about Chronic Lymphatic Leukemia.

From our research and the stories from other people who have CLL, we believe the food you eat has a large effect on your body. The people we talked with who are in remission almost all believe what you eat has a direct influence on this disease, CLL.

However, health organizations have concluded in their reports as of 2016 that there is no connection between diet and this disease.

Respectfully, we disagree with this conclusion and this is the purpose of our book. We believe diet has a lot to do with CLL and want to share how we came to this conclusion.

CHAPTER 1—CLL

Chronic Lymphatic Leukemial—Let's just call it CLL. This is a cancer of the white blood cells. The white blood cells are made in the marrow of the bones.

I have CLL and I want to share my journey with you in order to help you discover important information that will not be supplied by doctors and medical providers. So please stay with me. First I will provide basic information.

First, what is leukemia?

It is a malignancy (cancer) of blood cells. When you have leukemia, your bone marrow produces abnormal blood cells rather than regular blood cells. Most leukemias affect the production of white blood cells which are the cells that fight infections. Abnormal cells don't do the job they are supposed to. The leukemia cells continue to multiply, eventually forcing out the normal blood cells and the body loses its ability to fight infections, control bleeding, and transport oxygen.

There are different kinds of leukemia. The type depends on a few different elements. The speed of the progression and the type of blood cells affected determine the main category they fall under.

The four most common classifications are acute lymphocytic

leukemia, chronic lymphocytic leukemia, acute myeloid leukemia, and chronic myeloid leukemia. The function of all of these white blood cells when healthy is to fight infections. The different name types only need to be known by doctors and scientists. And a patient needs to know which one they have so they can work with the doctors on the best path of treatment in order to recover.

Acute lymphocytic leukemia (ALL) is the one most children get, but it also affects adults. This is the one the public has usually heard about. In ALL immature lymphoid cells multiply rapidly in the blood. This is caused by some DNA mutation but it is still unknown what causes the mutation to begin.

Acute myeloid leukemia (AML) involves the rapid growth of myeloid cells. It occurs in both adults and children.

Chronic lymphocytic leukemia (CLL) is a slow-growing cancer of lymphoid cells that usually affects people over 55 years of age. It almost never occurs in children or adolescents. CLL is called the "old man's disease" because more older men are affected than women.

Chronic myeloid leukemia (CML) primarily affects adults. It is slow growing and affects the myeloid type white blood cells.

Less common types of leukemia account for about 6,000 cases of leukemia each year in the U.S.

Leukemia is called an acute leukemia if it develops rapidly. Large numbers of leukemia cells accumulate very quickly in the blood and bone marrow, leading to symptoms such as tiredness, easy bruising, and susceptibility to infections. Acute leukemia requires fast and aggressive treatment or death will occur, generally within months.

Chronic leukemias develop slowly. Often they aren't diagnosed until symptoms appear, which doesn't occur until the number of white blood cells increase. If left untreated, the cells eventually grow to high numbers, and as in acute leukemias, cause similar symptoms.

I am 88 years young and almost an old man and the doctors say I have the "old man's disease* or CLL.

CHAPTER 2—THE BEGINNING OF MY CLL
GULFPORT, MISSISSIPPI

The cardiologist in the Gulfport ER was finishing my discharge paperwork while my wife and I waited to go home. Our visit was just another routine trip to the ER to deal with my high blood pressure and atrial fibrillation.

The ER physician glanced at the test results he had ordered. "Your white blood count is elevated. It should be 8,000-10,000, yours is 19,000."

Hmmm. Those numbers got my attention. On our next Biloxi VA appointment we told them about the elevated white blood count and we were referred to a hematology doctor for further testing. The hematology blood results came back and I learned I had Chronic Lymphatic Leukemia.

For months the VA doctors checked my lymph glands, and looked for bumps and rashes on my body. My white blood count rose to 30,000.

We were never advised what caused CLL or what to do to control the disease. I kept asking questions and not getting answers to satisfy my questions. The hematology doctor said my numbers were increasing by 5,000 per year. They prescribed 2,000 mg of B12 every day.

Cancer? Vitamins? I was concerned at the lack of information about this disease.

We moved to Alabama and had to select all new doctors. We researched specialists from two categories—civilian and V.A. in the area. We decided to base our decision according to their reputation. The civilian doctors were more accessible and were based in Fairhope, Daphne, Foley and Mobile. We needed a family doctor, a diabetes specialist, a cardiologist, a hematologist.

Also an eye doctor, as I now suffered inherited macular degeneration and was almost completely blind. And then an Ear/Nose/Throat doctor for reoccurring shingles in my ear, and a thyroid specialist, because my thyroid had been removed in Mississippi and now I also suffered from extreme dizziness

Strange how in such a short time I went from being in tip-top health to having so many multiple problems pouring down on me.

We were busy settling into our new home with doctor appointments scheduled almost every other day. It was hectic and unnerving.

I had operations on my eyes and my ears. I needed shots in my eyes every three months to slow the macular degeneration.

Two operation on my ears and I still became totally deaf in one ear.

Meanwhile, my white blood count soared to 50,000. And I

still took 2000 mg of B12 every day. Vitamins for cancer. Hmmm.

Within a few years my white cell count reached 65,000.

CHAPTER 3—WHY DO WE CONTINUE TO KILL OURSELVES?

Some health professionals become frustrated with their patients.

They try to heal us, and we continue to kill ourselves. Many doctors will not take you as a patient if you smoke. Some won't continue treatment if you refuse to lose weight through diet and or exercise. It is important to follow their orders if you want to get better. If you are overweight, have diabetes, and continue to eat a couple of donuts every day, why should they waste their time?

I knew Mickey Mantle, who drank and smoked. He died young at 63. He was famous for his words of wisdom during the last ten years of his life, "If I had known what this was doing to my body, I would have taken better care of myself."

Why do the doctors refuse to take you as a patient if you smoke? What does smoking have to do with our health? Why does second-hand smoke destroy the people near and dear to you? What is in cigarette smoke that kills us?

Of the more than four-thousand chemicals present in cigarette smoke, more than sixty have been identified as cancer causing chemicals, eleven are known to cause cancer in humans and eight others are suspected of causing cancer in humans.

These chemicals are considered toxic because they have

serious health impacts on the human body. For example: Hydrogen cyanide, carbon monoxide, and tar cause or are associated with cardiovascular disease and chronic obstructive lung disease; ammonia and formaldehyde cause eye, nose and throat irritations and other breathing issues.

Some of the toxins you have heard of: Nicotine, Formaldehyde, Ammonia, Hydrogen Cyanide (used in rat poison), Acetone, and Carbon Monoxide. One of the triggers for Leukemia? Benzene in the smoke.

For over 100 years, scientists have known that BENZENE is one of the elements in cigarette smoke and causes leukemia. Benzene is a clear, colorless, highly flammable and volatile, liquid aromatic hydrocarbon with a gasoline-like odor. It's found in crude oils and as a by-product of oil-refining processes. In industry, benzene is used as a solvent, as a chemical intermediate, and in the synthesis of numerous chemicals.

Exposure to this substance has been proven to cause neurological symptoms and affects the bone marrow causing aplastic anemia, excessive bleeding and damage to the immune system. Benzene is a known human carcinogen and is linked to an increased risk of developing lymphatic and hematopoietic cancers, acute myelogenous leukemia, as well as chronic lymphocytic leukemia.

Cigarette smoke is brought into our bodies three ways. Mainstream smoke, which is the smoke drawn in through the cigarette directly to the smokers lungs and nose. Second hand smoke which is exhaled by the smoker and inhaled by those in the area, and sidestream smoke which is the smoke from the end of a lit cigarette. All three methods deliver massive doses of toxins, including Benzene, a known trigger of leukemia.

It's all the same. If you are breathing cigarette smoke, you are breathing benzene.

Benzene , a clear, flammable, mobile, poisonous liquid obtained by scrubbing coal gas with oil, and by the fractional distillation of coal tar. It is used as a degreaser, a solvent and in the making of a vast number of every day products. They include plastics, insecticides, detergents, paints, dyes, perfumes and candles to name a few. The burning of tobacco releases Benzene into the air.

With an average of one non-smoker dying due to secondhand smoke exposure for every eight smokers dying of smoking related disease, it is no surprise that secondhand smoke is designated as a known human carcinogen (cancer-causing agent). Further, about half of regular smokers will die of a smoking-related disease and have a life expectancy of nearly sixteen years less than non-smokers.

The important fact is that cigarette smoking won't just harm you, it will likely harm your loved ones as well. And could even kill them.

CHAPTER 4—MORE ABOUT BENZENE

The chemical symbol for benzene is a six-sided hexagon and is our logo on the cover of our book. The symbol is over 150 years old and is still used today. it indicates an organic chemical formula for six-carbon atoms. The substance of benzene is called a hydrocarbon.

My first "introduction" to benzene occurred fifty years ago.

We passed the *Pizza Parlor* on our way home. We lived on Little Neck Road in Centerport, New York. The parlor was at the end of our street. We saw three men cleaning the *Pizza Parlor* floors. The lights were on and the men were mopping and degreasing the floors for the next day's business. Kitchens use a lot of grease and crews like theirs are hired to rid the restaurant of the grease.

Later that night we heard the fire house whistles and the engines sirens but we didn't see anything burning. The next morning we heard the news. The three men were dead. They used benzene to degrease the floors. One of the men lit a cigarette and the *Pizza Parlor* exploded. Benzene fumes are very flammable and explosive. Two of the men were found in the parking lot. They'd been blown out through the plate glass front windows. The third man was dead inside.

This story shows the highly volatile and flammable nature of benzene.

My research led me to learn as much as possible once I realized the same chemical that caused those deaths many years ago, might be partially responsible for my ailment.

Benzene is a pasty substance with a yellowish color and a pleasing sweet smell. It is highly volatile. A degreasing agent as described in the *Pizza Parlor* story, it is high in octane and therefore a valuable part of gasoline. Benzene in the gas keeps the engine from knocking.

Continual inhaling through smoke of any kind as well as breathing the fumes in a job that has high concentrations of benzene can lead to cancer, such as leukemia.

We found in our research that any smoke, whether it is from the fireplace, volcanoes, forest fires, fire pits, burning leaves, they all have benzene in the smoke.

If you smell gasoline you are inhaling benzene. The gas stations today are out in the open and some have air filters. If you smell gas, you are inhaling benzene. Some research even indicated some of the soft drinks have benzene. The plastic water bottles, any drink with vitamin C (ascorbic acid) plus either sodium benzoate or potassium benzoate can change into benzene when exposed to heat and/or light,

The Environmental Protection Agency, USA, classifies Benzene as a class A carcinogenic.

Benzene is everywhere and scientists have been aware of the dangers of benzene for over a hundred years.

The word "benzene" derives historically from "gumbensoin' (bezoin resin). European perfumers imported it from Southeast Asia back in the Fifteenth Century.

In 1825 the oily residue, derived from the production of illuminating gas, was given the name bicarburet of hydrogen. Scientists in 1833-1836-1845 first isolated benzene from coal tar. And benzene was discovered in deep space around 1997.

The carcinogen is present in many of the products we use every day in our homes and also in industries. Tires, rubber, plastic and gasoline are just a few. Long time exposure to benzene is known to cause anemia and leukemia. The anemia associated with benzene is aplastic anemia.

In the health organizations studies they have found a common cause of leukemia is benzene. Also among the studies we found CLL is often attributed to benzene from cigarette smoke.

At the end of many of those studies it states, "At this time there is no known connection between diet or smoking and CLL." I found this statement questionable since we KNOW benzene is a major factor and we read another report that suggested using the Mediterranean diet and the white blood cell count numbers will go down. I will follow up on our research on diet in a future chapter.

CHAPTER 5— HOW IS LEUKEMIA TREATED?

The acute leukemias need to be treated as soon as they are diagnosed. Treatment will depend on the age of the patient, the type of leukemia, how far it has advanced, and additional criteria. Aggressive treatment is usually needed to wipe out the deformed white cells.

Once remission is achieved, (usually five years without a reappearance) therapy may be continued to prevent a relapse. Acute leukemias can often be cured with treatment.

Chronic leukemias on the other hand are usually treated but not cured. Aggressive cancer killing treatment is often far worse for the human body than living with and controlling and managing the cancer symptoms of the chronic types. Some people with chronic leukemia may be candidates for stem cell transplantation, which does offer a chance for cure but is generally only used in more extreme cases.

CHAPTER 6—HOW IS CLL MEASURED?

A simple blood test. The lab tech draws tubes of blood from my veins and off to the lab they go. They are examined by a hematologist to determine what type of leukemia is present. The tests measure many things but our focus is on the rising white blood count. Every year mine increases by almost 5,000 WB cells. At least it was…

Christmas 2015, my white blood count was 65,000. That was my highest number. Now it is going down. Not because of the B12 vitamins. They had little effect. The only thing different in my daily life is…changing the food I eat.

The dramatic drop in numbers is a miracle to me. Other patients have had similar results.

I wasn't getting any helpful answers from my doctors, so I delved into exploring the massive studies related to Chronic Lymphatic Leukemia. Some of those studies stated there is no connection between our diet and CLL.

Yet friends and acquaintances who have CLL changed their diets and are in remission or at least lowering their white blood counts. We emphatically disagree with conclusions of the "studies."

We understand the scientists and researchers have a different threshold to meet to conclude that diet helps. That is why I am writing this book. I am not held to their criteria. I am only advising you of the results I have had and the results I have observed in friends and acquaintances. Some followed the Mediterranean Anti-Cancer Diet.

My status as an observer and victim of the disease leaves me the advantage of not needing to meet medical and legal restrictions or obligations. I am allowed to state my opinion and how I came to my conclusions without having to meet standards that can hinder helpful information.

Are you ready for action? Are you ready to fight CLL?

My first awareness as to how the food we eat relates to CLL begins with Mrs. Byrd and her family…

CHAPTER 7—A VISIT WITH THE BYRD FAMILY

My tenor saxophone was sold when we moved from Mississippi to Alabama. My friend gave me the name and address of the Byrd Family as they had a music store in their home. We stopped by to see if I could still play the sax while beset with all my medical issues.

While we were chatting a handsome young man arrived and Mrs. Byrd waved him over. "This is my son, George," she said.

He held out his hand. As we shook hands, I asked about his line of work.

"I am a Scientist" George replied.

Now my curiosity was aroused. You don't meet a lot of scientists. "What is your field of study?"

"The study of blood. I evaluate it in my lab."

Now I could hardly contain myself. "Remarkable, I've had CLL for ten years. My white blood cell count was at 65,000 and last week the VA called and told me my numbers are 57,000. A shocking drop of 8,000. I was pleasantly surprised, but also curious. Do you have any ideas as to why my numbers dropped so dramatically?"

George nodded. "My grandmother had CLL and she has recovered."

Mrs. Byrd smiled when the conversation turned to CLL. "My mother suffered from CLL for 20 years. Her white blood count was over 100,000. She recovered ten years ago and is now 96. Would you like to meet her?

"Mother's CLL numbers started to drop when she changed her diet ten years ago. She stopped eating bread and started eating green leafy vegetables and other seasonal vegetables. The cancerous white blood cell numbers started to go down. The cell numbers dropped until the numbers got down to the normal range of 8,000 to 10,000. She felt better as the numbers dropped to normal. That was ten years ago."

WOW! I never dreamed that leukemia could disappear on its own. Yet here is a lady who had CLL for 20 years and it has disappeared. She has been leukemia free for the last 10 years. She has many friends who are also better. Cured? Remission? Ready to return as active CLL? Is it possible?

After eleven years living with CLL, she was the first person with CLL I'd met who was in remission. It gave me hope.

CHAPTER 8—DIETARY CHANGE: A START TOWARD RECOVERY

The VA doctor called with the news that my white blood cell count dropped from 65,000 in January 2016 to 50,200 in September 2016. This drastic drop has given me hope that I might have found a path to a cure or remission.

If you have CLL, do NOT eat white bread. Eat vegetables, kale, broccoli, collards, turnips, bok choy. For a tasty treat, try cucumbers with the green skin on marinated in apple cider vinegar.

From the Farmer's Almanac: The old-fashioned farmer's medicine included four ounces of apple cider vinegar a day. It must be the *unpasteurized, organic apple cider vinegar with the mother of vinegar* (a type of fermenting agent).

If you eat a salad, be sure to use the apple cider vinegar. For hundreds of years, men have harnessed the benefits of apple cider for our health. It helps the body break down the nutrients in the salads, nutrients the body can absorb and use to heal. Be sure to purchase the unpasteurized apple cider vinegar with the mother label!

Calcium is vital for your body. It is for your bones. Besides leafy green vegetables, there are other sources to of calcium. Some seeds: sesame, poppy, and almonds are very rich in calcium. Legumes and beans are also good sources. Parmesan and other hard cheeses are loaded with calcium. Look for the fortified foods. Read the label. Orange juice and other fortified foods also have calcium. Take control of your food. Take a calcium pill if needed. Make sure you are getting a steady dose of calcium to keep your bones strong. CLL is a disease of the 'bone' marrow, so your bones are an important element in recovery, making calcium one of the most important elements in your recovery.

Our scientists discovered diphtheria was linked to drinking raw milk. The National Health Organization decided to protect the public from the diphtheria germ, and in the 1930's, the milk industry began pasteurizing our milk. Milk still has some of the calcium, but you know what happens when you heat milk? Most of the calcium benefits are destroyed in the pasteurization process.

CHAPTER 9—DIET TO HELP STENGTHEN BONE MARROW

Osteoporosis has to do with the density of the bones. Leukemia is the mutation of cells in the bone marrow.

The government changed its stance on osteoporosis and now says that diet can make the bone harder and stronger and healthier and slow or even reverse mild osteoporosis.

Calcium is a nutrient necessary for the growth and maintenance of strong teeth and bones, nerve signaling, muscle contraction, and secretion of certain hormones and enzymes.

Since calcium is known to help bones, it isn't a huge jump to think it might also help the bone marrow.

Below is a list of high calcium foods:

Dark leafy lettuce greens 1 cup chopped 41 mg (8% DV)
Okra 1 cup sliced (160g) 124 mg (12% DV)
Broccoli 1 cup chopped (91g) 43 mg (4% DV)
Low fat milk and yogurt 448 mg (45% DV)
Seeds: Seeds are tiny powerhouses. Some of them are high in calcium including poppy, sesame and celery.
Cheese: Most cheeses are excellent sources of calcium. Parmesan cheese has the highest calcium levels at 331 mg or 33% of the RDA per ounce (28 grams).
Low fat cheese (mozzarella nonfat) 1cup shredded provides 109 % RDA)

Fortified Soy products (Tofu) 1 cup 868mg (86% DV)
Green snap beams 1cup raw (110g) 41 mg (4% DV)
Almonds 1 cup whole (143g) 378 mg (38% DV)
Chinese cabbage (bok choy) 1 cup shredded (70g) 74mg (7% DV)
Fish canned: (Sardines, in oil, with bones) 1 cup drained (149g) 569mg (57% DV)
Sardines 1 can of sardines provides 35% of the RDA.
3 oz of canned salmon with bones have 21% of the RDA.
Edamame and Tofu Edamame are soybeans in the pod. 1 cup of edamame has 10% of the RDA of calcium.
Fortified drinks Non-dairy milk and orange juice can be fortified with calcium, 1 cup of fortified orange juice can have 50% of the RDA
Whey Protein Whey protein is an exceptionally healthy protein source. A scoop of whey protein power has 20% of the RDA for calcium,
Dark leafy greens 1 cup of cooked collard greens contain 25% of the RDA of calcium
Figs Dried figs contain more calcium than other dried fruits. A single ounce has 5% of your daily need for this mineral.

The government changed their position about diet and osteoporosis. They may eventually change their position on diet and CLL.

We aren't done yet. A calcium rich diet is part of the dietary change but our research brought us much further.

CHAPTER 10—OUR AMAZING BODY

Red blood cells, white blood cells and platelets are produced in the bone marrow, the soft fatty tissue inside the bone cavities. Just picture the marrow as a blood cell producer. During the production the blood stem cells in the bone marrow are programmed to make different types of blood cells.

Redblood cells: Carry oxygen through the blood vessels to the entire body.

White blood cells: Keep the immune system healthy, fighting off infectious germs and viruses.

Platelets: Tiny blood cells that coagulate the blood and form clots to prevent bleeding.

The bone marrow makes red blood cells at a rate of 2.4 million per second. That's right. I said 2.4 million per second. We truly do have an amazing body.

The blood cells do their job and then die off. When they do not die off or over-produce, they become too crowded. The crowding causes deformities, the cells no longer know how to carry out their purpose and the result is the weakening of the body.

CLL occurs when the white blood cells from the bone marrow greatly increase. Due to the excess cells and limited room, the cells start to change shape, become deformed, and change purpose.

This is the beginning of the white blood cells turning into cancerous cells and when this happens it develops into leukemia (CLL).

Blood thickness and coagulation is controlled by the platelets.

When the white blood cells become deformed and change purpose they invade the lymph glands, but most serious of all they weaken the immune system.

I have tried to find the magic cure. My white blood count was increasing and I am aging. As the count increases and attacks the immune system my body will not be able to fight off this CLL unless I can reverse those numbers.

The doctors look for the side effects from CLL: sleepiness, dizziness, chills, itching, or lumps over the body. If it increases to the point of attacking the liver and the spleen, doctors usually head for chemotherapy.

My big surprise was finding Mrs. Byrd, who changed her eating habits after having CLL for twenty years and drastically changed her numbers. She has been cancer free for ten years— or as the doctors say, "It is in remission."

One of the suggestions among my research was ingesting apple cider vinegar with the mother. A friend of mine gave me a big bag of green vegetables. They were mostly cucumbers. I soaked the slices of cucumbers in apple cider vinegar and ate them at every meal for six weeks. Rather tasty and good for me as well.

During that six-week period my white blood count numbers dropped from 57,000 to 50,200.

My German Grandmother Oma listened to the radio all day while working in her hand laundry business in 1930-1940. The programs she loved the most were Amos and Andy, Stella Dallas, Only The Shadow Knows and Dr. Frederick Carlson. His program and books were, "You are what you eat."

Many of his suggestions for a healthy life still hold true. "No smoking, use only apple cider vinegar instead of white vinegar, no white bread. Eat vegetables, especially dark green vegetables."

The Farmer's Almanac for one hundred years has said that two foods should always be in the kitchen cabinets, apple cider vinegar and honey. Using these products would help to keep you healthy. My Oma took this advice seriously and she lived to a very old age.

The only control we have is what we eat from birth to death. Our amazing body will do the rest.

CHAPTER 11—THE MEDITERRANEAN DIET— ANTI-CANCER DIET

The whole concept of an anti-cancer diet is to deprive cancer of what it needs to survive. Cancer is a hardy entity. It survives in an oxygen free atmosphere. It usually takes highly toxic chemicals to eradicate it from our system. It appears bionic, yet cannot last long without food.

Therein lies the logic behind the anticancer diet. Feed your normal cells, but deprive the cancer cells.

The Mediterranean Diet originated in Greece, Italy, and surrounding countries. Those cultures enjoy good health and live longer than people in other countries. The diet varies from country to country but basically kept the food natural and healthy.

The principal aspects of this diet include high consumption of olive oil, legumes, unrefined cereals, fruits and vegetables, moderate to high consumption of fish, moderate consumption of dairy products (mostly as cheese and yogurt), moderate wine consumption, and low consumption of red meat.

Studies have confirmed the Mediterranean diet lowers heart disease and lengthens life. Olive oil is considered the main ingredient in their healthy diet.

There is some evidence that regular consumption of olive oil may also lower the risk of cancer.

To follow the Mediterranean diet, first rid your kitchen of ALL processed foods. Do not purchase any more processed foods. Once you become accustomed to eating healthy fresh foods, you will probably not be tempted to return to the processed garbage. Fresh, unprocessed foods are so delicious and satisfying.

Avoid these foods: Refined sugars, refined grains, transfat, refined oils, processed meat and highly processed foods. See the picture? Refining, processing, adding unnatural preservatives harms our bodies.

The Mediterranean diet mentions the vitamins the fresh food provides and how the body uses these vitamins. Listed here are the vitamins that are needed to keep your immune system healthy and able to protect your amazing body.

VITAMIN A-helps to repair and regenerate tissues and aids in the absorption of iron.

VITAMIN E- an antioxidant that helps your body fight off infection.

VITAMIN B6- needed for adrenal function and is necessary for key metabolic processes.

VITAMIN C- aids immune function and helps provide protection against infections.

VITAMIN D - cell growth, promotes neuromuscular and immune function and reduces inflammation.

FOLATE-necessary for red blood cell development, low in folate makes the body more likely to develop cancer.

IRON-is a carrier for your body to carry oxygen to cells.

SELENIUM-helps the body to reject certain forms of cancer.

ZINC-controls inflammation and slows the immune response.

Recommendations from the Mediterranean diet even suggest you drink water and wine. Only fresh unprocessed fruit drinks without added sugar. Red wine, one glass is good, none if you have a problem with drinking. Coffee and tea in moderation.

Read the ingredients on the packages of the food you buy. You must take charge of what you are putting into your body. As the book says, "You are what you eat."

No smoking. No processed foods such as hot dogs, lunch meats. Use honey instead of white sugar. When you drop your guard on your eating habits, your immune system will be jeopardized.

Remember the Scarsdale Diet? In his book Dr. Scarsdale noted that 70% of the food in the grocery store is not fit for human consumption.

You should eat: vegetables, grain, whole grain breads, grain based pasta, rice, beans, nuts, legumes and seeds. Fish and seafood at least twice a week. Poultry, eggs, cheese and yogurt are also good for you. Avoid red meat. Eat dark chocolate, honey and brown sugar as Sweeteners. Avoid sugar in soda, candies, ice cream and granulated sugar. (Remember cancer cells love sugar.)

There is no special way to cook the above items, but all of the above are good and healthy. Know what you eat. Stick to it. Be healthy and enjoy your life.

CHAPTER 12—BETA-GLUCAN: THE FUTURE?

Diseases do not take hold in a healthy body. Our immune system is designed by our creator to fight off invading foreign germs so our body will stay healthy. My immune system was attacked and I now have CLL. This is leukemia. The white blood cells have become over crowded, changed shape. Because of this, my immune system cannot properly protect my body. The white blood cell count should be around 8,000-10,000. Mine is 50,200. My disease is, Chronic Lymphatic Leukemia.

Scientists have found a possible medicine in the cell walls of yeast, fungi and seaweed to help fight cancer. This medicine has been used in Japan, Taiwan, China and other countries. It is a natural substance. You can find more information on the search engines on your computer.

Scientists have been working with Beta-Glucan for over fifty years. For most of that time, it was so expensive the general public could not afford the medicine. But, not any more. We were shocked to read about Beta-Glucan. I just ran across it while researching information about CLL.

Beta-Glucan stimulates or restarts your immune system. There is much needed information about this treatment. Our scientific community in the USA is working on it. There are natural over the counter remedies as well as prescription strength. We are not suggesting that you run out and buy Beta-Glucan. Talk to your doctor about this addition to your treatment plan, another way of fighting cancer, then follow his or her instructions.

CHAPTER 13—CONCLUSION

My doctors tell me I stand a good chance of living ten more years. That would make me 98. They say this individually, but all use the ten year measure of the number of years.

The searching, reading, believing and not believing, uncovering information about our amazing bodies has been a very interesting and informative time of my life.

I never really understood why doctors didn't want you to smoke. Digging into this research has been eye opening as one subject led me to yet another. I now understand the danger of benzene.

One way of helping to destroy the cancer cells is to eat properly, like the anti-cancer diet and the Mediterranean diet. Another possible diet is the ketogenic diet. This research advises that cancer cells need eighteen times more sugar than non-cancer cells to grow and prosper. A ketogenic diet (one that generates ketones) consists of high protein, high fats and low sugar.

Another interesting part of this dietary study is that the brain can switch over to burning ketones to keep itself functioning, but the cancer cells can not. They must have simple sugars to survive.

In this summary of the study of leukemia, I want you to

know that white blood cells help fight infection by attacking bacteria, viruses and germs. The white blood count can inform you and your doctors about an undiagnosed medical condition. These blood cells are formed in the bone marrow, but go all over your body in the blood vessels.

CHAPTER 14—TELL ME YOUR STORY OF POSSIBLE REMISSION

My white blood count was 65,000. How high will it go? What is the maximum number? How will I know? The doctors have told me that they have seen patients with numbers of 150,000-200,000 and the patients were surviving nicely. So is 65,000 just the beginning? By lowering it to 50,000 and maybe more as I continue my diet, will I regain some of my strength?

CLL attacks the immune system. I watch for the side effects. The doctor's instructions are to wash my hands at least four times a day to keep the germs on the run.

There are others with CLL who have gone into remission. The medical profession cannot talk about nor give any information about their patients.

I have spoken to some other sufferers among ourselves who believe they have gotten their CLL under control. Some believe diet is one of the answers. Maybe diet change is the answer. Maybe it is Beta Glucan.

If you want to share your story about living with CLL and about your white cell numbers, if they go up or down, we'd like to hear your own story. We do NOT use personal information. Nothing will be published with your name on it, but maybe you can share information with others and help out another sufferer.

If you contact me, please note your white cell counts, their highs and lows, side effects you encountered, and what age you were when first diagnosed. Anything you think may have a bearing on your disease, please send it along.

What diet are you following? Has it made a change? Are you using apple cider vinegar and if so, how much daily? How much bread do you eat? Other carbs? We are interested in what you eat and the results you encounter. Are you taking vitamins? Maybe you can help us expand the nutritional information.
PLEASE SEND YOUR LETTER TO:
William and Carolyn Courduff, 14208 River Oaks Drive Foley, Alabama 36535
Or Email: bandccourduff@gmail.com or call: Home phone: 251-988-8684

If you provide a return address, we will notify you of the results and send you a copy of our new edition after we include the updates.

Before you do anything, we want to thank you for your interest in reading our viewpoint.

You have already participated in better health by thinking about, "You are what you eat."

Good doctors have been sent from heaven for me. Good doctors are why I am still here. Thank you.

~ Bill Courduff